Be Peace Now

an Infinite Light Transmission ™

a course for peaceweavers

the
course
and
journal

as transmitted to
Laurelle Shanti Gaia

Published by:

Infinite Light Healing Studies Center, Inc.

www.infinitelight.com

1-800-359-3424

Published in the United States of America.

Cover Design: Laurelle Shanti Gaia,
Infinite Light Productions
P.O. Box 1930
Sedona, AZ 86339

Illustrations: Joan Rudholm

Dedication

This book is dedicated to Gaia,
the living being that is our Mother Earth,
and to Divine Love, the only true power.

"Blessed are the Peacemakers, for they shall be called the Children of God"
Matthew 5:9

Acknowledgments

I thank my friends, my family, my spiritual teachers, and all the peaceworkers I have met along this path for helping to bring this course into the manifest plane.

Special thanks to James Lovelock for bringing to science what I feel in my heart; my parents for raising me to love, respect and honor the earth and Michael, Lynda, Janny, Julie, Matthew, Jessie, William, Joan, Gwen, Dennie, Beth, Vicky, Linda, Craigie, Lyn, Frank, Sandy, Dee, Elmina, Doug, Marilyn, Mari, Janeanne, Annie and Jerry, Utumei, Jesus, Chenrezi, Mikao Usui, Mother Teresa, Tiava, Lamaeha, Kalaelah, Ashaelah, Koteah, Mahone Nay, my special friends in Canada, Australia, Mexico, Italy, and Trinidad plus the countless others from around the world ... thank you for the love and the light that you are. Thank you for remembering with me, who we are and why we are here.

"Once we understand our full potential as powerful spiritual beings, we can focus this power on being peace, and healing our environment, our societies, and our planet."

Laurelle Shanti Gaia

4

Table of Contents

"You may say I'm a dreamer, but I'm not the only one

I hope someday you'll join us and the world will live as one"

John Lennon

Over the years I have come to know that peace isn't something that we need to search for, it isn't even something we need to "create" it is something that we all *are* inside.

Being peaceful is a choice that we can make. I find that it is easiest for me to be peaceful when I am living my life in a way that my needs are met, and when I am making a positive contribution to others.

There was a time that I thought I needed to make a positive contribution to others *before* I could consider my personal needs. I now understand that way of thinking contributes to the illusion of separation, which stands in the way of peace. *"Be Peace Now"* has helped me embrace my own Divine essence. The more we learn to embrace our personal Divinity, the more natural being peaceful becomes. Healing is the result of opening to our innate ability to be peaceful. *"Be Peace Now"* is a tool that helps us find that place of peace inside.

We are here on this planet to learn that it is actually very simple to *Be* Love and to *Be* Peace. We are here to awaken to the knowing that humanity has the power to live in peace, this very moment. Join me on a journey into the peace that you are.

Om Shanti Gaia
...Laurelle

"He who cherishes a beautiful vision, a lofty ideal in his heart, will one day realize it. Columbus cherished a vision of another world, and he discovered it, Copernicus fostered the vision of a multiplicity of worlds and higher universe, and he revealed it; Buddha beheld the vision of a spiritual world of stainless beauty and perfect peace, and he entered into it.

Cherish your visions, cherish your ideals, cherish the music that stirs in your heart, the beauty that forms in your mind, the loveliness that drapes your purest thoughts; for out of them will grow all delightful conditions, all heavenly environment, of these, if you but remain true to them, your will at last be built."

James Allen

Be Peace Now is a tool to help us create peace within our own hearts, and to share this with the world. It is based on these simple concepts; all things are energy, and energy is constantly changing. Every person on this planet is a powerful spiritual being and, in our own way, we are each affecting change.

Many people have experienced a demonstration of the reality that thought and prayer create change. Have you ever prayed for a sunny day for a special event, or used the power of positive thought to manifest the perfect parking place? These are basic examples of how we can create our own reality with our thoughts. . . so why limit this power?

Imagine what will happen when, daily, you use the power of the spoken word, prayer, and special energetic techniques focused to raise the peace vibration, and heal our Earth. Now imagine what will happen when millions, or billions of people around the planet do this too.

Be Peace Now contains a specific set of techniques that can be easily incorporated into our daily life to create peace consciousness and heal the Earth.

7

All over the world there are groups who meet to meditate and pray for world peace. This course is designed to enhance this work, empower it and accelerate healing and creation of, or awakening to peace.

This course, or program, is a spiritual healing practice designed for people of all religions, or of no religion. We all possess the Christed Consciousness, the essence of enlightenment, but most of us are not yet fully awake to it's full potential within us. This course can help awaken our dormant, enlightened, inner knowing. If the term Christed Consciousness causes you concern, I would ask you to reflect on the Divine Light that has been present in all avatars, i.e. Jesus, Buddha, Krishna, the Divine Mother; and know that this is what is meant by the term. I would ask you also to reflect upon the fact that all avatars delivered the message that we each carry within us this same Divine Light, the Christed Consciousness, the essence of enlightenment. These terms are synonymous.

This course has been developing for over forty years, and has grown out of a personal childhood experience. One summer, while on vacation with my family, I was playing in the Atlantic Ocean in Florida. I was pushed under the water by a wave, and was held under for what seemed to be eternity. Just as I began to panic, I was "inspired" to breathe very gently and not draw the water into my lungs, but to simply <u>ask</u> the oxygen in the water to help me breathe. I did exactly as I was told, and immediately became calm and peaceful.

I then saw a light growing gradually brighter and from this light a form came forth. I recognized this form to be Jesus, and suddenly he was surrounded by many beings that I could not identify at that time.

As this form appeared clearer to me, from his chest a bubble of light appeared. It was beautiful, shimmering and iridescent. The bubble burst, not like one would expect, but it burst slowly and gently and from it emerged a beautiful symbol. That symbol is Utumei, and is explained later in this course. He then spoke to me and said;

"Laurelle, remember, remember, remember.... with this we shall create peace".

In that moment I found myself standing up, unharmed and very happy to be alive.

I didn't think much of this experience for many years. However, powerful events in my life unfolded to teach me of energy, and the fact that we are all spiritual beings capable of emanating the full power of Universal, Divine healing love.

In 1994, I recalled the childhood experience very clearly and I began to receive light and energetic messages containing certain vibrations and information. One of the messages said that these were "transmissions of Infinite Light". I began to share this information, as I was guided, with people who I knew to be experienced with healing energies, prayer and the power of positive thought.

Every person who incorporated the transmissions into their personal lives, or their healing work, reported beautiful experiences of healing, spiritual growth and empowerment.

Many have found, that after exposure and integration of these energies, they became keenly aware of their personal "calling" in life. They were awakened to their latent abilities as artists, musicians, composers, healers, effective parents, inspirational speakers, etc. *Simply by allowing this energy into their lives, people are remembering who they are.*

In February of 1998 I was given the missing piece of information that I had longed to receive; the instructions on how this was to be used. This is a Course for Peace, for healing the Earth and increasing the frequency rate of the peace vibration on our planet. I was told when to teach the first class, what to teach and I was given a full course outline, and ultimately guided to write Be Peace Now.

I struggled with this a bit, fearing that perhaps I would not communicate it properly, or effectively and I didn't want to make a mistake or misinterpret something. This presented me with the opportunity to heal and remove the filters I was allowing to exist between my mind and the Divine mind.

The Infinite Light continued to move through me, helping me look at my insecurities and heal that egoic interference.

Because of this, I am now able to humbly offer this course to you with all my love. I have done my best to present these abstract concepts clearly, and it is my sincere prayer that you find it easy to follow and you are inspired to begin to use it to help heal our Earth and to become peace.

The Infinite Power of IAM

In this course, you will discover, that we use energy infused affirmation. Affirmations themselves, when they go against a core belief or our soul's wisdom are rarely effective. However, even affirmations that go against a core belief can be effective when infused with the full power of Divine Love and Light from the heart and the mind of God.

Our soul knows that we are all one within the heart and mind of God. This is where we are all perfectly whole and perfectly healed and we are connected as one united soul light. This is **The IAM**. IAM is the full power of divinity within all creation.

Therefore, when we begin any affirmation with "IAM" we are activating this infinite power of oneness from within the core of our being. You will find that the primary affirmations we use are;

IAM Infinite Light,
IAM Infinite Love,
IAM Infinite Peace,
and So IAM

Concepts of the course

"I would like you to come with me on a great adventure, an exploration
of humanity's potential as seen through the eyes of the planet,
and to share with me a vision of our evolutionary future.

"The journey will take us beyond this place and time, allowing us to
stand back and behold humanity afresh, to consider new ways of
seeing ourselves in relation to the whole evolutionary process.

"We shall see that something miraculous may be taking place
on this planet, on this blue pearl of ours. Humanity could be on the
threshold of an evolutionary leap, a leap that could occur in a flash of
evolutionary time, a leap such as occurs only once in a billion years.
the changes leading to this leap are taking place right before our eyes . . .
or rather right behind them, within our own minds."

Peter Russel, 1983

This course can help awaken our power to contribute to the healing of the Earth, raising the consciousness of humanity, and the co-creation of world peace. It is also heightening our awareness that we are all Divinely guided spiritual beings, and that through right use of this guidance we are limitless. The course is based on a 8 simple concepts:

1. All things are energy in one form or another.

2. Energy is simply light that vibrates at varying frequencies. The more rapid the vibration, the more light it contains. Peace is a vibration.

3. There is a collection of energy, known as the collective consciousness, which contains the essence of all conscious thoughts, past, present and future. This consciousness creates our perception of reality.

4. Every individual is personally *responsible* for the energy transmitted by their thoughts because they participate in the creation of the collective consciousness, and therefore we co-create our own reality.

5. Divine Light and Divine Love are the highest forms of energy and, when joined together, they become one transformational power.

6. *Every* individual has access to the full power of Divine Love and Divine Light.

7. We each have the power to positively affect the vibrational frequency of any person, place, or thing.

8. When individuals form groups for the purpose of accomplishing a goal, group consciousness develops which has an exponential effect on the goal.

Since the beginning of time we have been aware of two primary energy forms. We perceived them as light and darkness, positive and negative, good and evil. However, they are simply light and less light.

In the past, we have believed that we must have an equal balance of light and darkness. As we awaken to the Age of Peace the vibrational shift in consciousness is changing this paradigm. Our world is beginning to retain more light than darkness, so we can experience perfect peace as our reality.

To accomplish this people are needed, who are willing to take a few moments each day to help weave peace in their own hearts, into their lives and around the planet.

As we become peaceful in our own hearts, we align with our personal purpose for being alive, we remember who we are. As we are truly understanding that we are spiritual beings placed on this earth to remember our divinity, to understand that *the only true power is love* and to carry out the mission that the Creative Divine Consciousness is offering us . . . we are tapping into this power and transforming the world.

It is the power of the group consciousness that is going to bring peace to the planet, not one individual, not a "chosen one".

"There is a Light in this world . . .
a healing spirit much stronger than any darkness we may encounter.
We sometimes lose sight of this force . . . where there is suffering, too much pain.
And suddenly the spirit will emerge . . . through the lives of ordinary people
and answer in extraordinary ways."

Mother Teresa

"Our deepest fear is not that we are inadequate. Our deepest fear is that we are powerful beyond measure. It is our Light, not our darkness, that most frightens us. We ask ourselves: Who am I to be brilliant, gorgeous, talented and fabulous? Actually, who are you NOT to be? You are a child of God. Your playing small doesn't serve the world..."

Nelson Mandela

The Gaia connection

This course is based on the wisdom that all of creation is energy, and that Gaia is the living being we know as our planet Earth. Gaia is an energetic being with a physical, mental, emotional and spiritual body. She is affected by environmental, mental, and emotional toxins just as the human body is. Additionally Gaia is healed through the energetic balancing effects of spiritual healing, light transmissions and prayer energy.

The Gaia Hypothesis

"Our Planet ~ Mother Earth ~ is a Living Being and all life forms are her offspring."

The Gaia Hypothesis was formulated by Dr. James Lovelock, A British chemist specializing in atmospheric sciences. NASA requested that Dr. Lovelock and other researchers search for evidence of life on Venus and Mars. Through this research it became apparent that the Earth's atmosphere is unique within our solar system.

Dr. Lovelock considered the history of the Earth's evolution to be from an environment that supported the earliest life forms, small and simple beings that lived in the oceans and were less than a single cell. Gradually, the atmosphere shifted from a dominance of carbon dioxide, to a predominant mixture of nitrogen and oxygen, which began to create an atmosphere that would favorably support animals and humans

Could this mean that we, as Gaia's children are evolving as she is. Mother Earth creates from within her being all forms of life. Does this prove that God is in Gaia, and in her children?

"Is it not written in your law? I have said, 'You are Gods'"

John 10:34

Our body contains billions of cells working together as a single life form, just as billions of life forms on Gaia become a living super organism.

We can recognize the contribution of our seas and our atmosphere serving as Gaia's respiratory system sharing oxygen and carbon dioxide.

Gaia's circulatory system is comprised of our waterways and streams.

Our planet's meridians and nadis are invisible leylines moving through and around her body supporting her flow of life force energy.

As the moon contracts and expands it's gravitational force, so beats the pulse of Gaia and all who harmonize with her.

Humans who soul-resonate with Gaia find the cycles of their life aligning with the seasons of the year.

The Gaia Hypothesis was named for the Greek Goddess who drew the living world forth from Chaos. There is spiritual power in the sound of the name Gaia. Chanting it calls forth Gaia's IAM presence.

This healing IAM presence of our Earth Mother will assist us as we awaken from chaos to the Age of Peace.

As peaceweavers we are energetically impacting Gaia's healing. We are learning to dream with Gaia and visualize a world at peace with an abundance of resources, for all people.

A message from Gaia

"Welcome children of peace, I embrace you.

Thank you for hearing this message and opening your hearts, minds and souls to the energy upon and within these words. You are remembering your choice and I embrace you. You carry the peace ray within you . You hold the vision beyond the vision for you are the very essence of peace ...and you are remembering this.

Please pause for a moment and prepare to connect with the very essence of this message. You may begin by placing your focus upon your breath. Let it be deep, soothing, and calming. Allow yourself to begin to experience an expanded reality.

You may experience this by closing your eyes .... focus on your breath ... expand your awareness above you and around you ... intend to expand and become aware of your connection with the light of your soul . .. breathe into this awareness ... now expand more and become aware of the light of your soul group ... breathe into this connection .... expand and become aware of your connection to the full intensity of the Divine heart and mind...breathe into this expanded awareness. Allow the full intensity of this light to flow . . . from the heart and mind of the Divine ... into the light of your soul group ... expanding its light ... breathe ... next allow the expanded light of your soul group to flow into the light of your soul ... breathe ... increase the light of your soul ... and now allow the full intensity of this expanded light to flow into your energy field and your physical body ... flowing from above ... around and within ... breathe ... breathe ... breathe ... feel the intensity of the light you now hold.

You are here in this moment to make the most important choice that you can make in this lifetime. That choice is whether you will accept the power of Divine love that you are. This choice is whether you will continue to accept that which you perceive to be darkness, or whether you will come to know that darkness is simply the conscious limitation of love. You have the choice to release the distraction of focusing on that which is not real, and to shift your focus to the Divine in all things.

You may choose to see peace as light. When you choose to BE that light of peace . . . peace will BE. It is that simple, for the Divine is not complicated and the Divine is unlimited. The frequency that is peace is stronger than all the darkness that some perceive to be exploding on the earth.

I am the voice of mother earth, and I am the soul of reality.

Please know that which is not real is simply less than the full power of the light of Divine love. It is not truly dark, it is not evil, yet it is awakening light.

See my children ... See. See the waring, see the terror, see the pain as awakening light. See the transformational potential in this awakening and hold the great vision . . . hold the vision beyond all limits.

The great vision calls you ... it calls all light workers ... it calls all peaceweavers to this purpose. The purpose is to be who you truly are, to be the light of peace and to place your focus always upon the light of Divine love which resides in all people, all actions, all things. Light is awakening within even that which appears to be the darkest of the dark . . . and you each transmit the light that awakens ... you do this by being peace.

The intensity of Divine light is expanding ... the volume of light is increasing. This is the focus ... This is what you see .... the rest is invisible. Perhaps you will you will see the irony ... what humanity has perceived to be invisible is visible through the eyes of the soul. In the text of your Bible you find the Christed one of that time, the one known as Jesus to say:

Jhn 20:29 Blessed are they that have not seen, and yet have believed.

You may ask ... have I felt peace within myself ? Can I see peace in the same way as I can see war ? If you have felt peace within yourself ... yet have not "seen" peace ... you still know that peace is very real. You see the invisible with the eyes of your soul. Together you have the power to awaken humanity to the age of peace. You have the power to transform the collective creative God consciousness by raising the frequency of the peace ray with your thoughts, words, visions and actions. As one prophet of peace implored you ... so do I implore you .... "Be the peace you want to see in the world."

"As we attune to Gaia's dreamspace, we assist her in holding a vision of perfect peace and we anchor the peace ray into the heart of the Earth"

Laurelle Shanti Gaia

Participation in the course

This is the first of several phases of this work. This book contains the information needed to establish the foundation for amplification of the peace vibration within the participant, or "peaceweaver".

There will be a variety of ways to participate in this course, this book is one. It is also possible to attend a workshop to participate in demonstration and practice of this energy work. The Be Peace Now Audio Program is available to provide audio support. Details are available on page 140 of this manual.

This first phase includes symbols which are transcendental in nature, and assist in helping the peaceweaver create an energetic connection with specific streams of energy contained within the peace vibration and to integrate these frequencies into their body.

As a participant, you will be introduced to the symbols and their purposes, and some basic information about the human subtle energy system as it relates to this course. You will then learn to create a sacred space from which to do this work.

The first phase of the course is divided into sections that include a series of meditations, affirmations, and mantras. These are done daily for a prescribed period of time, and then the peacemaker moves onto the next set.

The sets can be done in less than 10 minutes a day, and require no special tools or environment. *However, consistent daily practice is imperative.*

If you must interrupt the process for some reason and skip a day or more, you will begin again from the start. When this happens, it is simply the way the energy itself insures that we, as peaceweavers, are integrating and anchoring the energies effectively. It is not an indication of weakness, or failure. It only means that, for some reason more of the introductory level energy needs to be anchored. This could be for the participant personally, or perhaps it is to help pace the collective group energy. Remember, there are many people around the planet doing this work, and the energy that we each are contributing is affecting the whole.

23

When you have completed the entire phase as prescribed, you will then be ready to move to the next phase.

There is also a journal page supplied for each day to record your experiences. This is an important part of the program. Be sure to record what you experience during the meditation, and also at the end of your day, make notes of things that happened during the day. Often as our vibration shifts to a different frequency we begin to notice energy we exchange with others through communication or another form of interaction, produces different results than before. We also may find ourselves more in tune with synchronistic events which can guide us through our day. We become more aware of the miracle that each day is.

It is important to complete the exercises exactly as prescribed because the vibrational alteration in the peacemaker's energy takes place only by moving the energy as directed, and for the required period of time. This change empowers the peaceweaver to emanate and transmit higher levels of the peace vibration. So as one moves through the course, they will transmit increasingly higher frequencies of light.

As you begin this journey into the energetic recreation of our world as we know it, let me thank you for hearing this call. Your participation, at whatever level you choose, is acknowledged and appreciated. You are an instrument of peace and healing by the simple act of reading this and allowing your consciousness to flow and merge with the peace stream.

"We cannot live only for ourselves. A thousand fibers connect us with our fellow men; and among those fibers, as sympathetic threads, our actions run as causes, and they come back to us as effects."

Herman Melville

Our subtle energy system

Our bodies, and Gaia's, are much more than the physical forms that we are familiar with. We also have an etheric energy field, which consists of spiritual, mental and emotional layers, woven into a cocoon of light. It is this cocoon of energy that houses our life force. We also have energy centers, or chakras, which act as valves for life force energy to flow in, around and through.

Chakra centers of energy align the human body's biological systems and link them with the external energy fields. When the centers are purified, and vibrationally accelerated they create network portals for sending and receiving light.

This illustration represents the primary chakras utilized in the course, with the Stellar and Gaia gateways creating portals which anchor and seal in high frequency light.

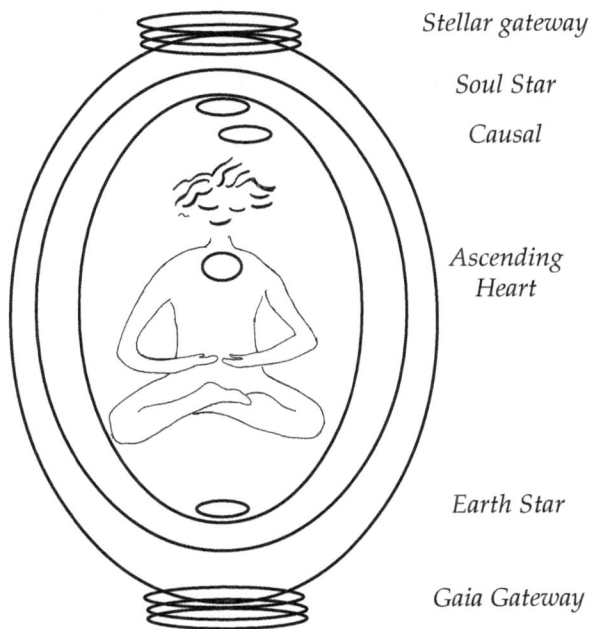

Stellar gateway

Soul Star

Causal

Ascending Heart

Earth Star

Gaia Gateway

We will not address the biological functions of the chakras here. Our focus is on chakra functions as they relate to peacework. You will learn more of this as you move through the daily practice.

The Ascending Heart chakra helps us hold higher frequencies of light when it is activated. *The Ascending Heart is the Power center for the Age of Peace.*

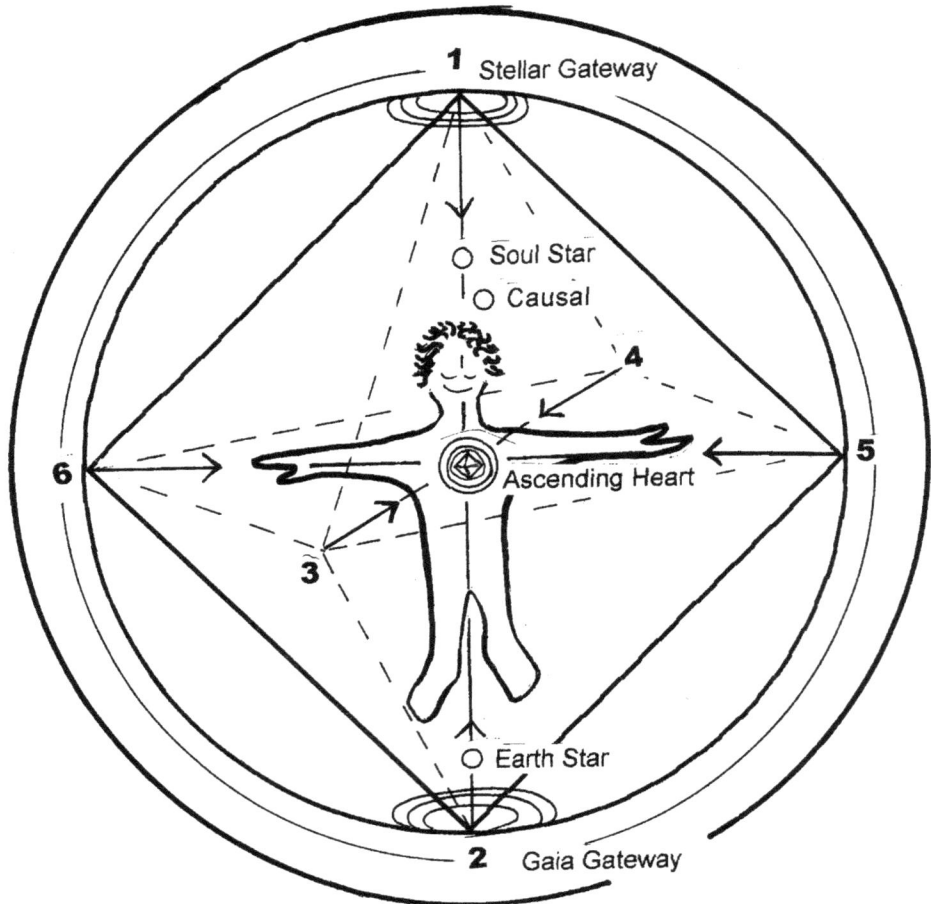

In these exercises we will learn how to activate the Ascending Heart, which contains the personal essence of our Godself. We will use this to create a sacred space, within which to work.

"When you feel overwhelmed ... or do not know what to do next, take one step at a time . . . look before you in the moment and say, '

What is it . . . that I have to offer?
What is it . . . that is burning inside of me?'
What is that ember of light . . .
that is trying to blaze forth and illumine the world?

You each hold this ember.
You each are the light of peace"

~ Utumei

The symbols

Symbols have been used in healing, and spiritual practice throughout history. The symbols used in this course are transcendental in nature, meaning they are connected directly to the Divine consciousness. Each symbol is a representation of a unique vibration, and creates a specific effect.

The symbols introduced here are Altea, Anye, Utumei, and Om Shanti Gaia.

Altea (ahl-tay-ah) ~ Sacred Space Creation

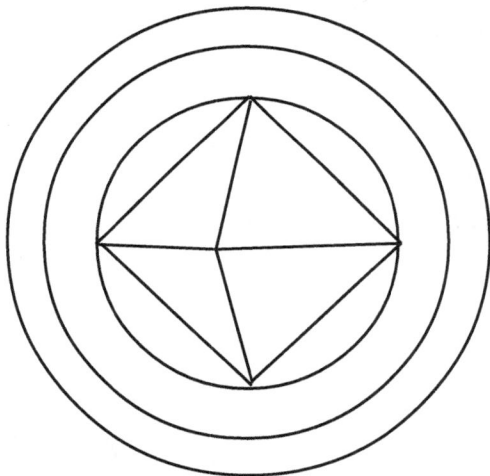

This symbol creates an octahedron (double, 4-sided pyramid) of golden light around the peacemaker. By activating the symbol at the ascending heart center, golden light flows and expands to create a golden octahedron of light surrounding all of the participant's bodies.

Utilizing Altea creates a strong energy field which has the power to completely and perfectly integrate energies contained within it. When one is sealed within this sacred space only high frequency light can exist within the chamber. All light energy work done in this space is enhanced.

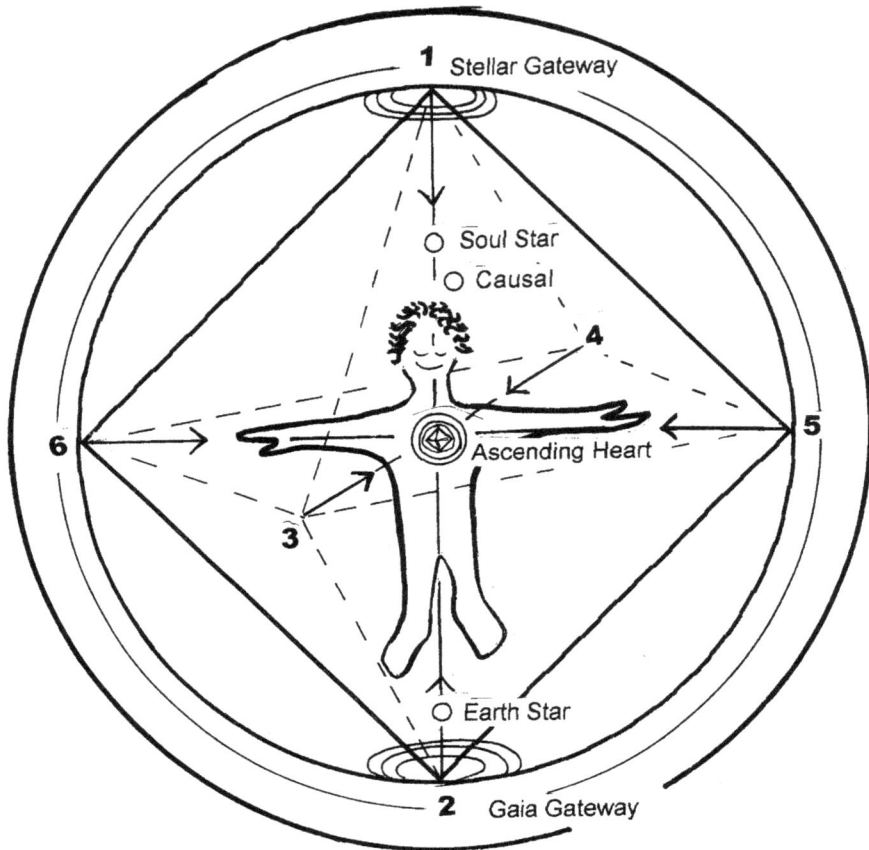

Each pyramid, in this application, has a four-sided base. The bottom pyramid is inverted with the apex passing through and connecting just beyond the Gaia Gateway, the top pyramid is upright with the apex passing through and connecting just beyond the Stellar Gateway.

The base of each pyramid intersects the ascending heart, and the essence of the symbol Altea remains active at this energy center. Once activated a sacred chamber of high frequency light is created.

Anye (ahn yay) Aligning Heaven and Earth

Anye aligns the soul star with the earth star, allowing perfect integration of the Divine essence of stellar and earth energies within the human energy system. It has a grounding effect much more suitable to a participant of this course than meditations or techniques that connect one strongly to the earth energy only.

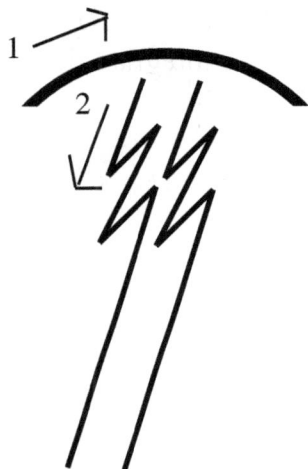

Utumei (oo-too-may) The Essence of Enlightenment

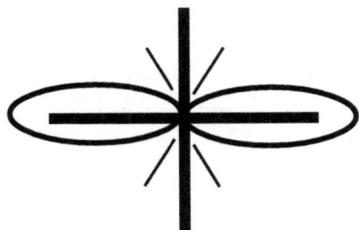

Utumei is the symbol of the Christed Consciousness, Divine Light, the essence of enlightenment.

Use of this symbol assists in release of egoic interference to the integration and acceptance of our personal Divine power. Utumei helps us dissolve the veils of fear; fear of being all that we truly are.

Om Shanti Gaia activates the essence of peace within the soul of Gaia. This symbol facilitates the peacemaker's ability to dream with Gaia and help awaken humanity to perfect peace as our reality. As the family of Gaia, the peaceful essence of our souls is activated from within as we integrate the emanations of Om Shanti Gaia.

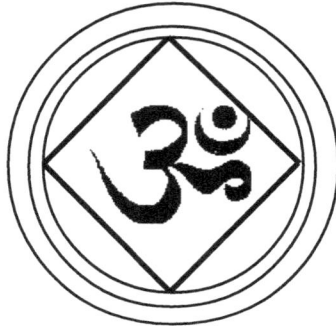

Om Shanti Gaia

Fear is the greatest obstacle to peace. Fear of not having power, fear of not having enough food, water, clothing, land, work, etc. Fear is at the root of anger , greed, illness and war.

When we realize that we can collectively create a world of abundance, by simply sharing the resources we have, and learning to live in harmony with our Earth, we can transform fear into peace.

Fear is simply lack of love, and where love is lacking, peace cannot prevail. There are specific exercises in this course that are designed to transform fear by infusing the fear vibration with the high frequency light of love.

"The ultimate purpose of the Infinite Light Transmissions is the manifestation of perfect peace within all of creation.

Now is the Time."

~Utumei

Daily peace sessions

This course includes illustrations and instructions for daily Infinite Light peace sessions, as well as journal worksheets to record your thoughts, feelings and experiences.

In addition to the basic content of this course, a key factor to the success of this work is sacred intention, and Divine command.

Marcel Vogel, an IBM researcher stated that intent produces an energy field, and our thoughts and emotions affect living things around us.

Sacred intention is focused thought, communicated from the center of one's soul to their Divine creative intelligence. Sacred intention is stated with simplicity and clarity, and is further empowered when spoken in the form of a prayer of gratitude for the manifestation of the intention.

Divine command is claiming of one's own power of creation through focused thought from the brain frequency known as the theta state. In theta state our brain waves slow to 4-7 cycles per second. This is the state used in hypnosis. As I am writing this my brain waves are are cycling at 14-28 cycles per second and I am in beta state. When one practices the daily peace sessions, theta state can be attained at will, which empowers the sacred intention and Divine command.

Prior to beginning the daily peace sessions it is suggested that each peacemaker form their personal sacred intention and state it in the form of prayer and Divine command.There is also an exponential effect when each of us, who participates in this course, offers the same prayer. The following is the example that many are using.

"Thank you Creator that ... that this sacred prayer is the Divine command for perfect peace for all creation . Thank you that there is complete harmony among all people now. Thank you for this prosperous world where all resources are shared peacefully and joyously. Thank you that humanity's consciousness is harmonized with Gaia now. Thank you that we give back to her as much as we take. Thank you that we care for Gaia, and all life with deep love." And So It Is

"Many who will be drawn to this course have a soul level sense of urgency for needed world transformation. Some may have become complacent by feelings that this is an insurmountable goal.

Some may have become scattered by focusing their energies in a multitude of directions trying to heal everything and mastering nothing.

These are manifestations of less light attempting to divert humanity from our Divine purpose. The way to overcome this diversion is through commitment to regular spiritual service" ~ Utumei

The Infinite Light peace sessions are a series of energetic activations, which allow us to infuse high vibrational frequencies of light into our physical and etheric bodies simultaneously. As we are able to hold these higher frequencies of light we become more peaceful within, and more aligned with our purpose in life. This allows us to live more as our higher self, or our "Divine self". Imagine a world where all people are living as their higher self!

Many healing forms or spiritual practices such as Reiki involve energetic attunements or activations in the form of transmissions passed from one person who has been empowered to do so to one who wishes to receive. These forms contribute greatly to the spiritual evolution of humanity, and are among the keys to moving into the Age of Peace.

Infinite Light peace sessions differ from these age old practices in that the peacemaker receives activations of their energy system, directly from the Divine, by simply practicing the daily peace sessions.

It is important for participants of this course to realize that from time to time very intense vibrational changes take place instantaneously, which may create strong sensory impressions. These can take many forms such as; sensing color or sound, feeling energy moving through the body, feeling warm, or cold, feeling "tingles", or the sensation that waves of energy or light are passing through you. Some people are less sensitive to the sensation of the energy and may not feel these things, which is normal as well. The goal is not to experience the "phenomena", it is to participate daily and allow growth to take place.

Those who do experience sensations may, at other times, feel as if nothing is happening. When we reach a certain frequency within the activation process, the energy shifts to the function of sealing the light into the bodies rather than continuing to increase the vibrational rate. As this sealing process is taking place it cannot be perceived by most people. *Know that the energy is continuing to work, but it is working on a higher level than we can discern with our physical senses. Once the sealing is complete, and daily practice continues, amplification of the frequency will begin again*

It is important to maintain the commitment to regular practice during these times.

To experience the maximum vibrational change, it is important to do the sessions daily. However, the Divine energy that is weaving the stream of peace as we work, may, from time to time guide us to stop for a day, a week, or longer. If this happens, don't be discouraged. Remember you are one of many people who are helping to create this tapestry of peace, and the energy balance is key. There is a larger picture here than any of us can see at this time. If you are guided to stop for any reason, do so. When you feel ready to start again, you must do so from the very beginning. By doing this you are helping to strengthen the foundation for peace.

The practices illustrated in this section include working with the symbols and energy, meditation, affirmation, and chanting. When we participate in daily peace sessions, it will take 11 weeks to move through the course the first time. Here is what you will do each day of the designated week:

Week 1
Prayer/sacred intention
Create the sacred space
Session 1

Week 2
Prayer/sacred intention
Create the sacred space
Session 2

Week 3
Prayer/sacred intention
Create the sacred space
Session 3

Week 4
Prayer/sacred intention
Create the sacred space
Session 4

Week 5-11
Prayer/sacred intention
Create the sacred space
Combination sessions

When you have finished this course, the initial energetic attunements will be complete. You can begin again and go all the way through the program, to move yourself to the next level.

There is great healing power in sound. Chanting specific mantras has been done throughout the ages to raise vibrational levels to reach higher states of consciousness.

The primary chant used in this work is "Om Shanti Gaia". Om being the power of the Infinite Divine Love which guides our universe. Shanti means peace, and of course Gaia is the living being that is our mother Earth.

When we chant "Om Shanti Gaia" we are invoking the full power of Infinite Love, the essence of peace and offering this to the earth.

You will notice at the close of each of the sessions we chant "Om Shanti Gaia" for at least three minutes. The longer you chant, the higher the vibration becomes, and the more positive, loving, peaceful healing energy you offer out into the collective consciousness. So chant for as long as you feel guided, and notice how you feel as you do this. When you are out in nature, you may notice that the chant takes on a different quality.

Om Shanti Gaia was offered initially with the Infinite Light Transmissions. It was reinforced one day during personal sacred ceremonial practice in the center of Stonehenge. As I meditated with the altar stone I began to hear it chant "Om Shanti Gaia" to me. It was as if I was hearing chants that transcend time and space as we perceive it. Every time I chant now I feel a resonance with that altar stone at Stonehenge.

You may chant "Om Shanti Gaia" as a guttural, or ancient sounding chant, or it may become songlike. Let it take whatever form feels right for you in the moment. If you don't like your "singing" voice, this is an opportunity to heal that perception. You will find, as you are doing these sessions, you become an instrument for spiritual energy to move through. If you will set your ego, or fears aside and simply let the *energy* flow through your voice, you may be very pleasantly surprised at the sounds you produce.

Let's begin by learning the process for creating sacred space, and the components of each of the sessions. First we will explore how we create sacred space by using our first symbol, Altea.

The exercise described on these two pages precedes *every* peace session. It can also be used anytime you wish to create a sacred space for meditation and healing, or raise the light vibration of any situation.

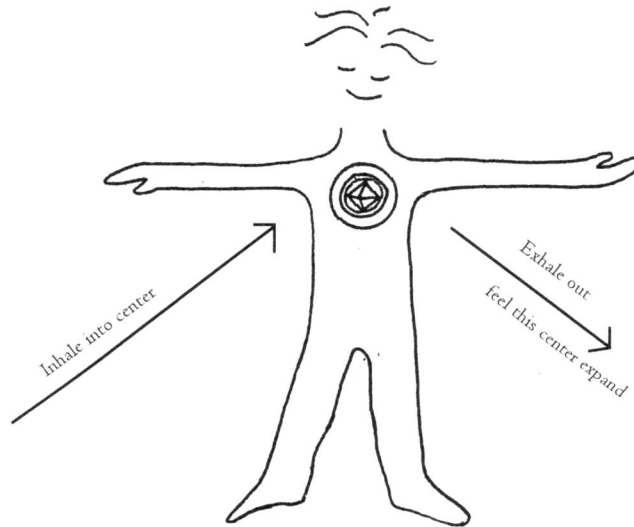

Stand with legs shoulder width apart, (or sit in lotus position) arms extended left palm facing up and right palm facing down.

Do three deep ascending heart breaths. Do this by forming the intention, or imagining that when you inhale you bring the breath into your ascending heart, and exhale from the ascending heart.

Feel Altea within the ascending heart - chant Altea in 6 sets of 3 as it expands and encompasses your whole body. ***This process "Sets the Altea Space".***

1. Altea~Altea~Altea . . . anchors stellar gateway apex

2. Altea~Altea~Altea . . . anchors Gaia gateway apex

3. Altea~Altea~Altea . . . anchors front point

4. Altea~Altea~Altea . . . anchors back point

5. Altea~Altea~Altea . . . anchors left point

6. Altea~Altea~Altea . . .   anchors right corner

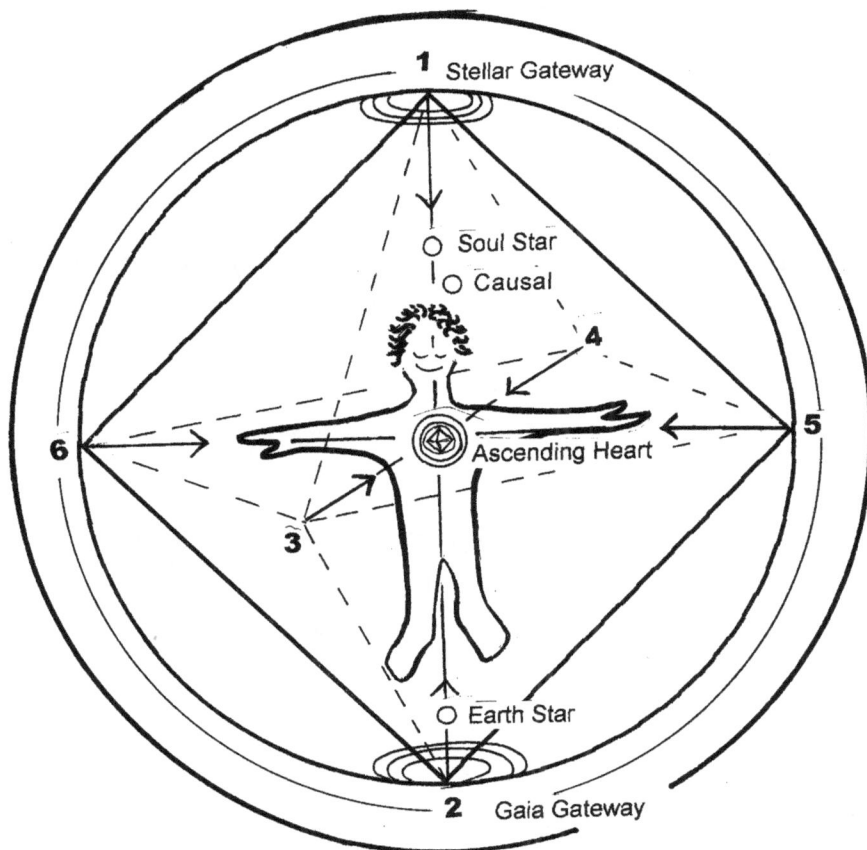

Stellar Gateway

Soul Star

pearlescent/opalescent white

Anye

silver gold

Earth Star

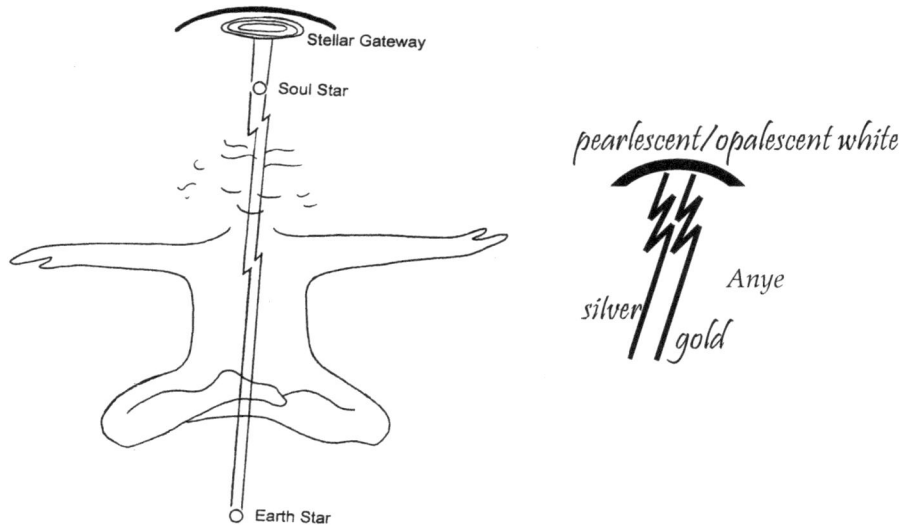

Begin by creating the sacred space as described on the previous pages. Next sit comfortably, feel the golden octahedron and spheres that cocoon you in your sacred chamber.

Bring Anye into your sacred space with the ***pearlescent/opalescent white*** arch over your stellar gateway and the streak of light in ***silver and gold*** moving through your soul star all the way to the earth star. Do this with visualization, or intending and thinking of the process.

Affirm 3 sets of the following:

I am Divine Alignment
I am Gaia's Nurturance
I am Divinely Guided Power

And So IAM

Chant *"Om Shanti Gaia"* for at least 3 minutes

Begin by creating the sacred space described previously. Next sit comfortably in the space you have created.

Draw Utumei in the air in front of you visualizing or imagining it as silver light. As you draw it say

"Utumei, Utumei, Utumei; as within so without, ALL are ONE".

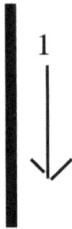

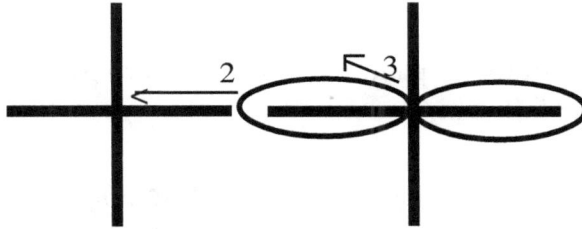

Draw infinity symbol
3 times and say
"Utumei, Utumei, Utumei"

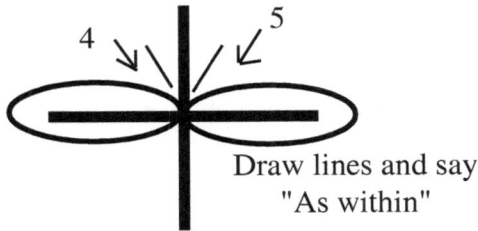

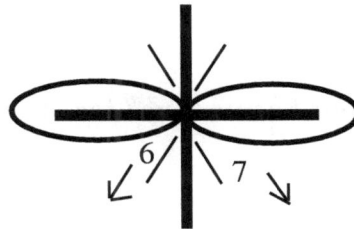

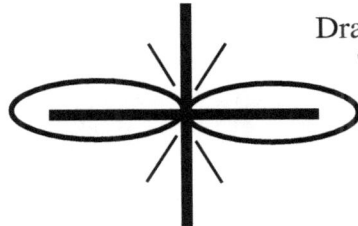

Draw lines and say
"As within"

Draw lines and say
"So without"

Beam a flash of light from the
palm of your hand to the center
of the symbol and affirm
"All are one". *continued on next page*

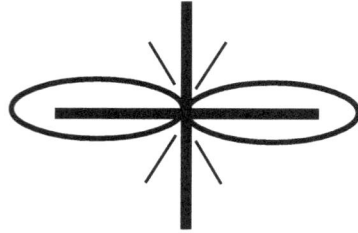

See and feel Utumei expanding and filling the space you are sitting in. Affirm 3 sets of the following :

I Am Infinite Light
I Am Infinite Love
I Am Infinite Peace
And So AM

Chant *"Om Shanti Gaia"* for at least 3 minutes.

Begin by creating the sacred space described previously. Next chant Om Shanti Gaia 15 times, 5 on each hand, using the mudra as illustrated. 5 times on the left hand . . .repeat on 5 times on the right hand ... then 5 times with both hands.

1. Open palm wide ... chant "Om"
2. Thumb touches index fingertip chant "Shan"
3. Thumb touches fire fingertip chant "ti"
4. Thumb touches ring fingertip chant "Gai"
5. Thumb touches little finger chant "a"

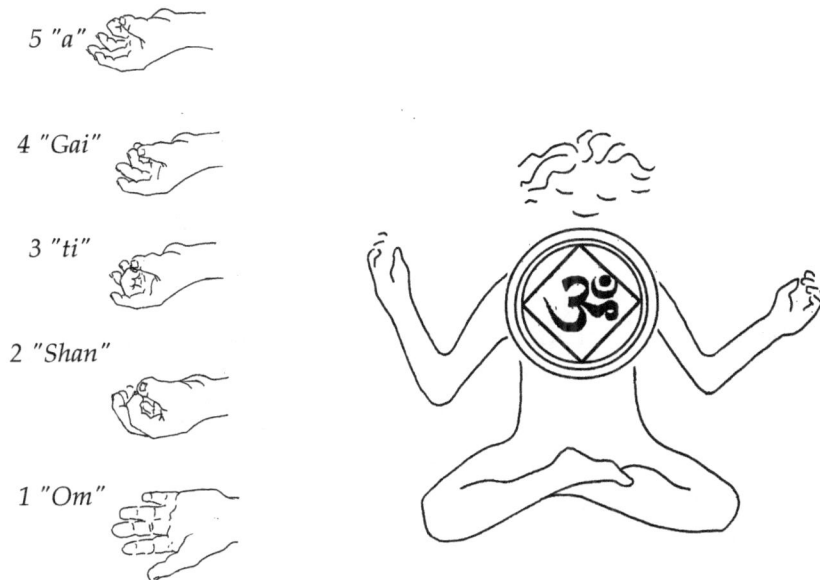

5 "a"

4 "Gai"

3 "ti"

2 "Shan"

1 "Om"

Next hold palms out and visualize or think of a multi-dimensional image of the Om Shanti Gaia symbol, superimposed over a vision of the Earth. "See" this between your hands. Energize it between your hands as you chant *"Om Shanti Gaia"* for 3 minutes or longer.

47

Begin by creating the sacred space described previously

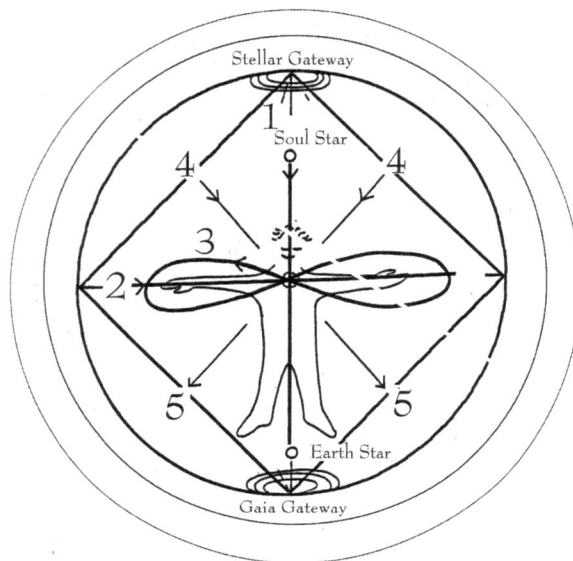

Call Utumei into your body in silver light, bringing in the energy with the following sequence:

1. Vertical beam of light from the stellar gateway through the Gaia gateway.
2. Horizontal beam of light from right to left.
3. Infinity ribbon of ***aquamarine light*** (see illustration on next page) from ascending heart out the front left, around to the back left, through the front, around to the right, enter into the ascending heart at the back . . . the infinity ribbon flows through 3 times as you say: *"Utumei, Utumei, Utumei"*

Next visualize diagonal beams of light (#4 in illustration) moving into the ascending heart as you say: "As Within"

Visualize diagonal beams (#5 in illustration) flowing from the ascending heart as you say "So Without".

48

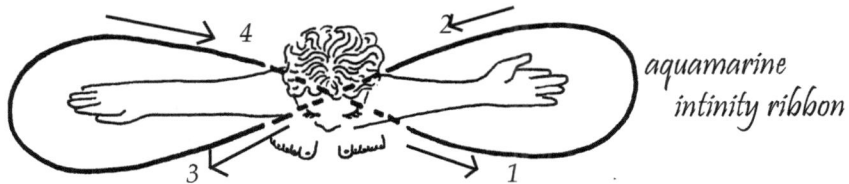

View of flow of ribbon of light from overhead.

The **aquamarine** infinity light ribbonflows horizontally, beginning at the ascending heart moving out the front, around to the left, enters the ascending heart from the back, passes through and flows to the right around to the back and enters the ascending heart again . . . repeats two more times.

Now sit in the sacred space you have created. With left palm facing up and right palm over your ascending heart , allow the golden light that surrounds you to flow into your left palm. Feel this light flow through and out your right palm. Beam the light into your ascending heart center with your right palm. Continue with the affirmation by saying *"All Are One"*.

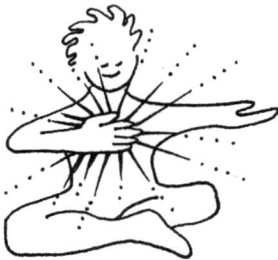

To close imagine Utumei and Altea blending with your ascending heart center. Place both palms over your ascending heart and continue to beam light into your being as you chant:

"Om Shanti Gaia" for a minimum of three minutes.

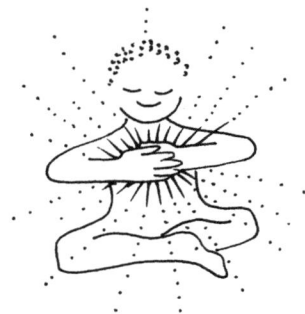

Journaling your peace sessions

Journaling your Infinite Light peace sessions is a key element to your progression through the course.

The following pages include quick graphic references to the sessions, for each day of the week during the initial 11 week program.

Make notations in your journal of any sensory experiences you had, i.e. what did you feel, see, or hear? Did you have any particular thoughts arise.

How did you feel when you started the session? Were you tired, rested, stressed, calm, angry, happy, etc. How did you feel when you completed the session?

What is going on in your life that is of particular importance at this time?

How are you relating to your family, friends, co-workers, and yourself? If any relationships are particularly difficult, or good, make a note of that. As you you begin to hold more light, you will notice the energetic exchange between you and those you regularly relate with may change. You will become more likely to attract better, higher forms of relationships, transform existing ones, or move on to healthier situations.

What are your personal goals for growth, healing and inner peace? Write them down, and watch how the energy helps you move closer to manifesting the goals that are truly in alignment with your life purpose.

Have fun with your journal be BOLD. You can write in it, draw in it ... color the pictures ... there are no rules ... express yourself! Grow! EnJOY!

pearlescent/opalescent white

Stellar Gateway

Soul Star

silver | gold

Earth Star

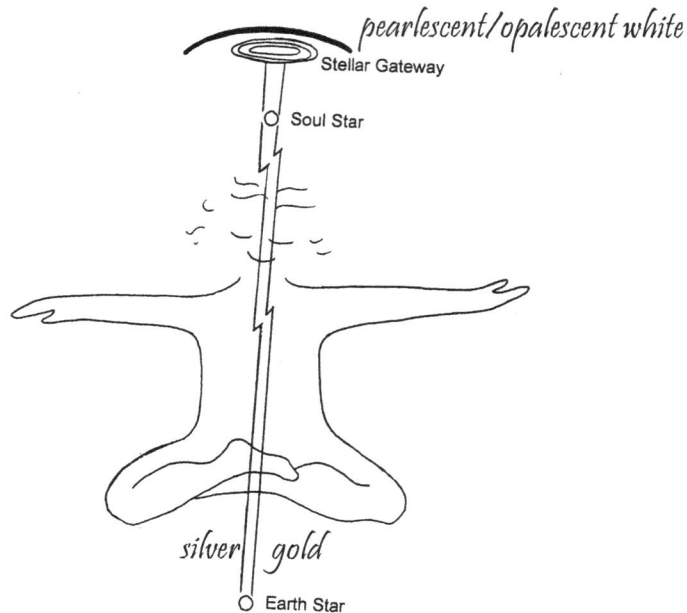

At a Glance - Session Summary
Do daily for 7 days
Set Sacred Intention/Prayer
Set the Altea space (page 38-39)
Anye (An-yay) - Imagine it moving through you

Affirm ~ repeat set 3 times
I AM Divine Alignment
I AM Gaia's Nurturance
I AM Divinely Guided Power
And IAM

Chant: "Om Shanti Gaia" for at least 3 minutes

When thought, purpose and prayer come together ... all things are possible

Date:_____ Time:_____

Location: _____

_____

_____

_____

_____

_____

_____

_____

_____

_____

_____

_____

_____

_____

_____

_____

Date:_____ Time:_____

Location: _____

_____

_____

_____

_____

_____

_____

_____

_____

_____

_____

_____

_____

_____

_____

_____

Date:_____ Time:_____

Location: _____

_____

_____

_____

_____

_____

_____

_____

_____

_____

_____

_____

_____

_____

_____

_____

Date:_____ Time:_____

Location: _____

_____

_____

_____

_____

_____

_____

_____

_____

_____

_____

_____

_____

_____

_____

_____

_____

Date:_____ Time:_____

Location: _____

Date:_____ Time:_____

Location: _____

_____

_____

_____

_____

_____

_____

_____

_____

_____

_____

_____

_____

_____

_____

_____

When the power of love overcomes the love of power
the world will know peace.
Jimi Hendrix

Date:_____ Time:_____

Location: _____

_____

_____

_____

_____

_____

_____

_____

_____

_____

_____

_____

_____

_____

_____

_____

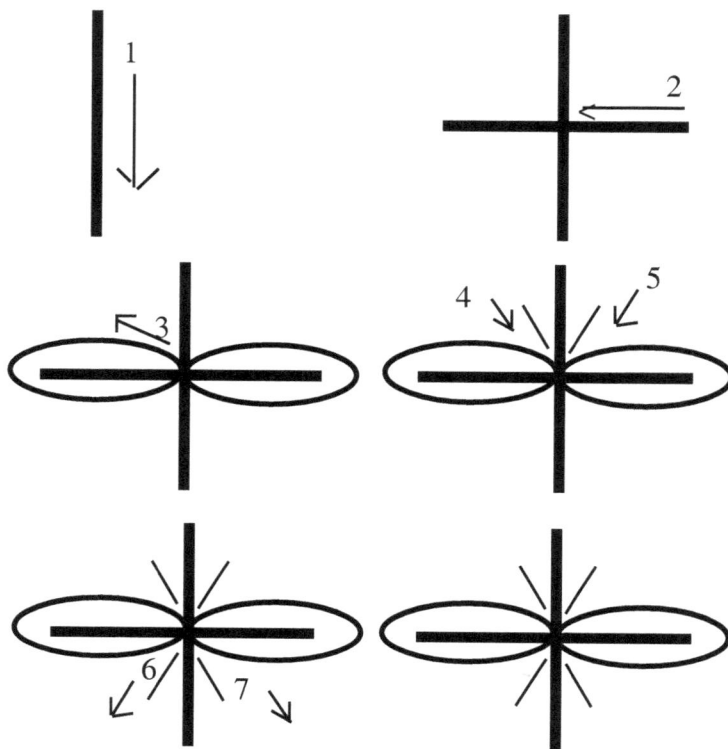

At a Glance - Session Summary
Do daily for 7 days
Set Sacred Intention/Prayer
Set the Altea space (page 38-39)
Utumei (oo-too-may) -
Imagine it as silver light filling the space you are in
Say "Utumei, Utumei, Utumei; as within so without, ALL are ONE".

Affirm - repeat set 3 times
I AM Infinite Light
I AM Infinite Love
I AM Infinite Peace . . . And So I AM
Chant: "Om Shanti Gaia" for at least 3 minutes

Allow the limitless light of your soul to flow into your heart
. . . bathe yourself in the essence of peace

Date:_____ Time:_____

Location: _____

_____

_____

_____

_____

_____

_____

_____

_____

_____

_____

_____

_____

_____

_____

_____

_____

Date:_____ Time:_____

Location: _____

_____

_____

_____

_____

_____

_____

_____

_____

_____

_____

_____

_____

_____

_____

_____

_____

_____

Date:_____ Time:_____

Location: _____

_____

_____

_____

_____

_____

_____

_____

_____

_____

_____

_____

_____

_____

_____

_____

_____

Date:_____ Time:_____

Location: _____

Date:_____ Time:_____

Location: _____

Date:_____ Time:_____

Location: _____

_____

_____

_____

_____

_____

_____

_____

_____

_____

_____

_____

_____

_____

_____

_____

_____

For some of us, the most effective way to develop inner happiness and peace is through religious practice. For others it may be non-religious practices. What is important is that we each make a sincere effort to take our responsibility for each other and for the natural environment we live in seriously.

His Holiness The Dalai Lama

Date:_____ Time:_____

Location: _____

_____

_____

_____

_____

_____

_____

_____

_____

_____

_____

_____

_____

_____

_____

"a"

"Gai"

"ti"

"Shan"

"Om"

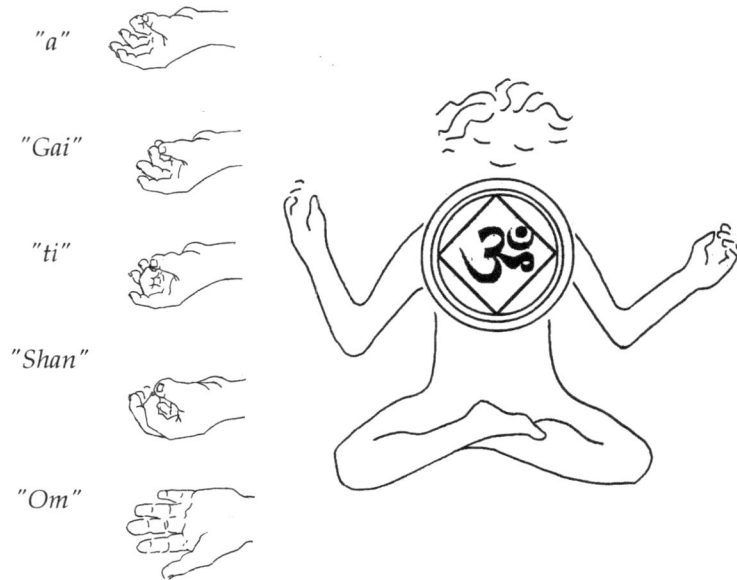

At a Glance - Session Summary
Do daily for 7 days
Set Sacred Intention/Prayer
Set the Altea space (page 38-39)
Om Shan ti Gaia mudra/chant 5 times on each hand . . .
left hand first then right

Hold your palms out . . . visualize or imagine a multidimensional
Om Shanti Gaia between your hands . . . energize it while you chant
"Om Shanti Gaia" for at least 3 minutes

Hold a vision in your heart . . . cherish it . . .
allow your dreams to take perfect Divine form

Date:_____ Time:_____

Location: _____

_____

_____

_____

_____

_____

_____

_____

_____

_____

_____

_____

_____

_____

_____

Date:_____ Time:_____

Location: _____

_____

_____

_____

_____

_____

_____

_____

_____

_____

_____

_____

_____

_____

_____

_____

Date:_____ Time:_____

Location: _____

_____

_____

_____

_____

_____

_____

_____

_____

_____

_____

_____

_____

_____

_____

_____

_____

Date:_____ Time:_____

Location: _____

_____

_____

_____

_____

_____

_____

_____

_____

_____

_____

_____

_____

_____

_____

_____

Date:_____ Time:_____

Location: _____

_____

_____

_____

_____

_____

_____

_____

_____

_____

_____

_____

_____

_____

_____

_____

Date:_____ Time:_____

Location: _____

_____

_____

_____

_____

_____

_____

_____

_____

_____

_____

_____

_____

_____

_____

_____

_____

_____

Imagine all the people living life in peace. You may say I'm a dreamer, but I'm not the only one. I hope someday you'll join us, and the world will live as one.

John Lennon

Date:_____ Time:_____

Location: _____

_____

_____

_____

_____

_____

_____

_____

_____

_____

_____

_____

_____

_____

_____

_____

Infinite Light Meditation ~ Journal
Aligning with the Divine Mind ~ Session 4
At a Glance - Session Summary
Do daily for 7 days

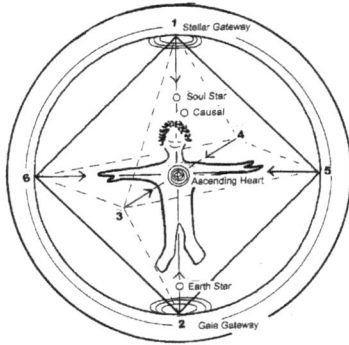

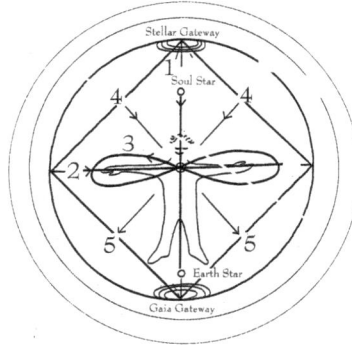

Set Sacred Intention/Prayer
Set Altea Space (page 38-39)

Invoke Utumei

1. Vertical beam of light

2. Horizontal beam

3. Infinity Ribbon

   Utumei, Utumei, Utumei

4. Diagonal beams in "As Within"

5. Diagonal beams out "So Without"

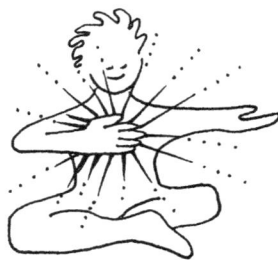

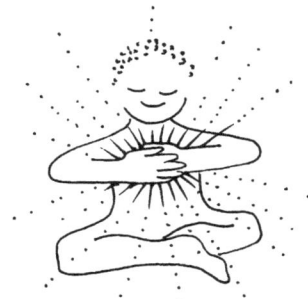

Left palm up - receive light
Right palm over ascending heart
beaming light in and affirm:
"All Are One"

Breathe Utumei and Altea into the
ascending heart. Place both palms over
ascending heart beaming light in as you
chant: *"Om Shanti Gaia"* for 3 minutes
or more.

Everything we achieve is a direct result of our own thoughts
... We each are an integral part of the Divine Mind.

Date:_____ Time:_____

Location: _____

_____

_____

_____

_____

_____

_____

_____

_____

_____

_____

_____

_____

_____

_____

Date:_____ Time:_____

Location: _____

Date:_____ Time:_____

Location: _____

_____

_____

_____

_____

_____

_____

_____

_____

_____

_____

_____

_____

_____

_____

_____

_____

Date:_____ Time:_____

Location: _____

_____

_____

_____

_____

_____

_____

_____

_____

_____

_____

_____

_____

_____

_____

_____

Date:_____ Time:_____

Location: _____

_____

_____

_____

_____

_____

_____

_____

_____

_____

_____

_____

_____

_____

_____

Date:_____ Time:_____

Location: _____

True peace is not merely the absence of tension: it is the presence of justice.
Martin Luther King, Jr.

Date:_____ Time:_____

Location: _____

_____

_____

_____

_____

_____

_____

_____

_____

_____

_____

_____

_____

_____

_____

_____

_____

Peace sessions weeks 5~11

Now that you have experienced all of the peace sessions, we will combine components from each of them, into one set that will be done daily for the remainder of this process.

It will be helpful for you to continue to journal your experiences, with as much detail as possible. Remember to make notes about changes in your relationships, your thoughts, feelings, and the way you perceive world situations, and your personal life purpose.

As we become more in alignment with our life purpose, we realize that our awareness is unfolding like the petals of a flower, as we are blossoming into our full spiritual potential on Earth. We rarely have an awareness of the "whole plan" that we are to accomplish. But we are learning to quiet ourselves from within and tune into the inner whisper that is available to guide us through our experiences. We move step by step and day by day as the plan reveals itself to us.

It is this gentle growth of our spirit that makes life a beautiful adventure, when we to be fully appreciate each life experience for its challenges as well its joy.

The dreamers are the saviors of the world.
Humanity cannot forget its dreamers; it cannot let their ideals fade and die;
it lives in them; it knows them as the realities which it shall see one day.
Composer, sculptor, painter, poet, prophet, sage, these are the makers of the afterworld . . .
the architects of heaven.

James Allen

pearlescent/opalescent white

Stellar Gateway

Soul Star

silver | *gold*

Earth Star

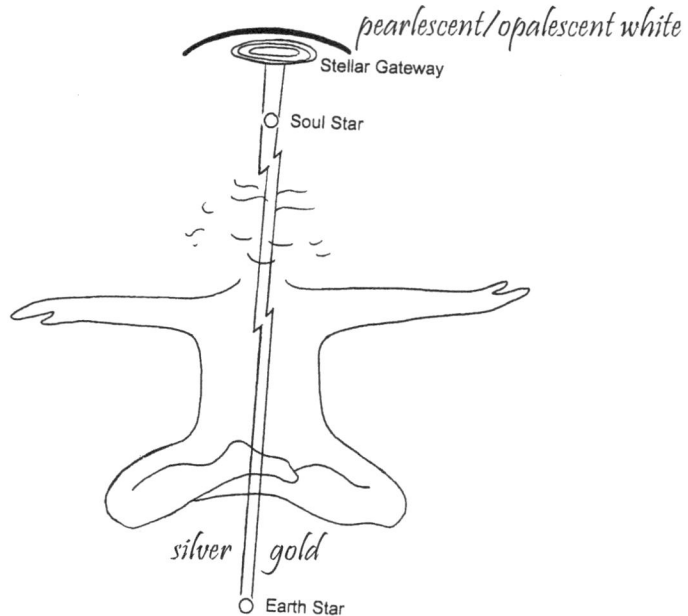

At a Glance - Session Summary
Do daily during weeks 5-11
Set Sacred Intention/Prayer
Set the Altea space (page 38-39)
Anye (An-yay) - Imagine
light moving through you

Affirm - repeat set 3 times
I AM Divine Alignment
I AM Gaia's Nurturance
I AM Divinely Guided Power
And So I AM

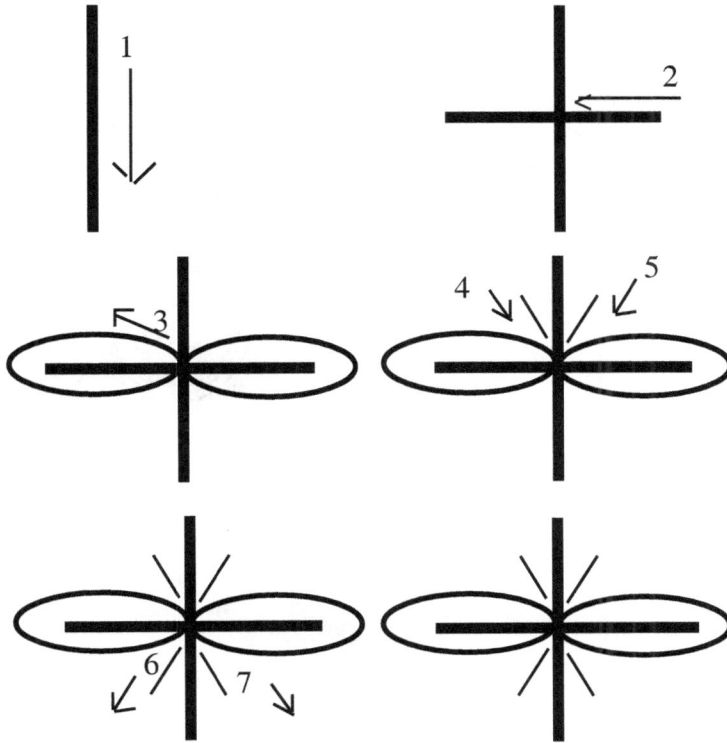

At a Glance - Session Summary
Do daily during weeks 5-11
Set Sacred Intention/Prayer
Set the Altea space (page 38-39)
Utumei (oo-too-may) -
Imagine it as silver light filling the space you are in

*Say "Utumei, Utumei, Utumei; as within so without,
ALL are ONE".*

*Affirm - repeat set 3 times
I AM Infinite Light
I AM Infinite Love
I AM Infinite Peace . . . And So I AM*

"a"

"Gai"

"ti"

"Shan"

"Om"

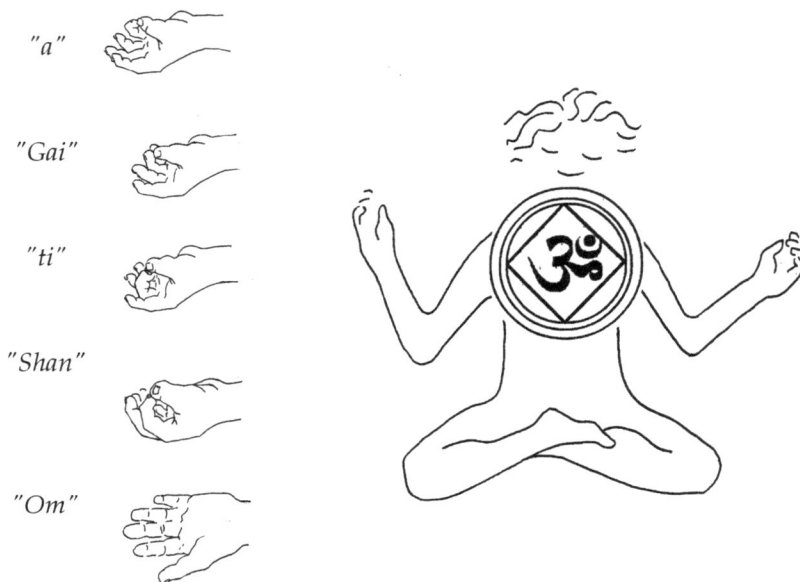

At a Glance - Session Summary
Do daily for during weeks 5-11
Set Sacred Intention/Prayer
Set the Altea space (page 38-39)
Om Shan ti Gai a mudra/chant 5 times on each hand . . .
left hand first then right

Hold palms out . . . visualize or imagine a multidimensional   Om Shanti Gaia between your hands . . . superimposed over an image of the Earth. . . . energize the vision while you chant

"Om Shanti Gaia" for at least 3 minutes

At a Glance - Session Summary
Do daily during weeks 5-11

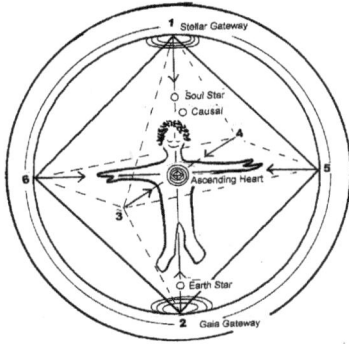

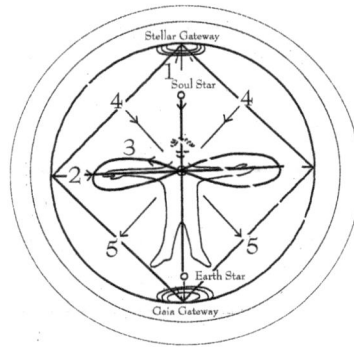

Set Sacred Intention/Prayer
Set Altea Space (page 38-39)

Invoke Utumei

I. Vertical beam of light

2. Horizontal beam

3. Infinity Ribbon

   Utumei, Utumei, Utumei

4. Diagonal beams in "As Within"

5. Diagonal beams out "So Without"

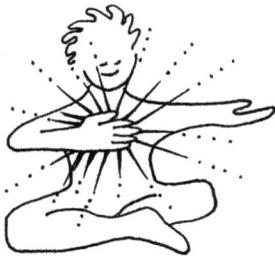

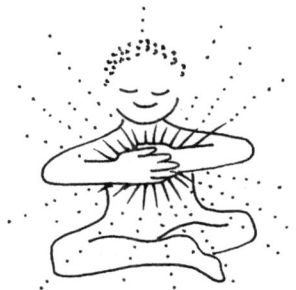

Left palm up - receive light
Right palm over ascending heart
beaming light in and affirm:
"All Are One"

Shrink Utumei and Altea into the
ascending heart. Place both palms over
ascending heart beaming light in as you
chant: *"Om Shanti Gaia"* for 3 minutes
or more.

89

When we move thru the veils of illusion, we recognize . . .
within the hearts of the Peacemakers . . . the Age of Peace is Now!

Date:_____ Time:_____

Location: _____

_____

_____

_____

_____

_____

_____

_____

_____

_____

_____

_____

_____

_____

_____

_____

Date:_____ Time:_____

Location: _____

_____

_____

_____

_____

_____

_____

_____

_____

_____

_____

_____

_____

_____

_____

_____

_____

Date:_____ Time:_____

Location: _____

_____

_____

_____

_____

_____

_____

_____

_____

_____

_____

_____

_____

_____

_____

_____

Date:_____ Time:_____

Location: _____

Date:_____ Time:_____

Location: _____

_____

_____

_____

_____

_____

_____

_____

_____

_____

_____

_____

_____

_____

_____

_____

_____

Date:_____ Time:_____

Location: _____

_____

_____

_____

_____

_____

_____

_____

_____

_____

_____

_____

_____

_____

_____

_____

One day we must come to see that peace is not merely a distant goal we seek,
but that it is a means by which we arrive at that goal.
We must pursue peaceful ends through peaceful means.
Martin Luther King, Jr.

Date:_____ Time:_____

Location: _____

_____

_____

_____

_____

_____

_____

_____

_____

_____

_____

_____

_____

_____

_____

_____

If I have been of service, if I have glimpsed more of the nature and essence of ultimate good, if I am inspired to reach wider horizons of thought and action, if I am at peace with myself, it has been a successful day.

Alex Noble

Date:_____ Time:_____

Location: _____

_____

_____

_____

_____

_____

_____

_____

_____

_____

_____

_____

_____

_____

_____

Date:_____ Time:_____

Location: _____

_____

_____

_____

_____

_____

_____

_____

_____

_____

_____

_____

_____

_____

_____

_____

_____

Date:_____ Time:_____

Location: _____

_____

_____

_____

_____

_____

_____

_____

_____

_____

_____

_____

_____

_____

_____

Date:_____ Time:_____

Location: _____

_____

_____

_____

_____

_____

_____

_____

_____

_____

_____

_____

_____

_____

_____

_____

Date:_____ Time:_____

Location: _____

_____

_____

_____

_____

_____

_____

_____

_____

_____

_____

_____

_____

_____

_____

Date:_____ Time:_____

Location: _____

_____

_____

_____

_____

_____

_____

_____

_____

_____

_____

_____

_____

_____

_____

_____

_____

There is a wonderful mythical law of nature that the three things we crave most in life . . . happiness, freedom, and peace of mind . . . are always attained by giving them to someone else.
Peyton Conway March

Date:_____ Time:_____

Location: _____

_____

_____

_____

_____

_____

_____

_____

_____

_____

_____

_____

_____

_____

_____

_____

We shall find peace. We shall hear angels. We shall see the sky sparkling with diamonds.
Anton Chekov

Date:_____ Time:_____

Location: _____

_____

_____

_____

_____

_____

_____

_____

_____

_____

_____

_____

_____

_____

_____

_____

Date:_____ Time:_____

Location: _____

_____

_____

_____

_____

_____

_____

_____

_____

_____

_____

_____

_____

_____

_____

_____

_____

Date:_____ Time:_____

Location: _____

_____

_____

_____

_____

_____

_____

_____

_____

_____

_____

_____

_____

_____

_____

_____

Date:_____ Time:_____

Location: _____

_____

_____

_____

_____

_____

_____

_____

_____

_____

_____

_____

_____

_____

_____

_____

_____

Date:_____ Time:_____

Location: _____

_____

_____

_____

_____

_____

_____

_____

_____

_____

_____

_____

_____

_____

_____

_____

_____

Date:_____ Time:_____

Location: _____

_____

_____

_____

_____

_____

_____

_____

_____

_____

_____

_____

_____

_____

_____

_____

_____

Nothing can bring you peace but yourself. N
othing can bring you peace but the triumph of principles.
Ralph Waldo Emerson

Date:_____ Time:_____

Location: _____

_____

_____

_____

_____

_____

_____

_____

_____

_____

_____

_____

_____

_____

_____

_____

Peace has to be created, in order to be maintained. It is the product of Faith, Strength, Energy, Will, Sympathy, Justice, Imagination, and the triumph of principle. It will never be achieved by passivity and quietism.

Dorothy Thompson

Date:_____ Time:_____

Location: _____

_____

_____

_____

_____

_____

_____

_____

_____

_____

_____

_____

_____

_____

_____

Date:_____ Time:_____

Location: _____

Date:_____ Time:_____

Location: _____

_____

_____

_____

_____

_____

_____

_____

_____

_____

_____

_____

_____

_____

_____

Date:_____ Time:_____

Location: _____

_____

_____

_____

_____

_____

_____

_____

_____

_____

_____

_____

_____

_____

_____

_____

Date:_____ Time:_____

Location: _____

_____

_____

_____

_____

_____

_____

_____

_____

_____

_____

_____

_____

_____

_____

_____

Date:_____ Time:_____

Location: _____

_____

_____

_____

_____

_____

_____

_____

_____

_____

_____

_____

_____

_____

_____

_____

Peace is not the absence of war; it is a virtue; a state of mind;
a disposition for benevolence; confidence; and justice.
Spinoza

Date:_____ Time:_____

Location: _____

_____

_____

_____

_____

_____

_____

_____

_____

_____

_____

_____

_____

_____

_____

_____

. . . peace is the climate of freedom.
Dwight D. Eisenhower

Date:_____ Time:_____

Location: _____

_____

_____

_____

_____

_____

_____

_____

_____

_____

_____

_____

_____

_____

_____

_____

Date:_____ Time:_____

Location: _____

_____

_____

_____

_____

_____

_____

_____

_____

_____

_____

_____

_____

_____

_____

_____

Date:_____ Time:_____

Location: _____

_____

_____

_____

_____

_____

_____

_____

_____

_____

_____

_____

_____

_____

_____

Date:_____ Time:_____

Location: _____

_____

_____

_____

_____

_____

_____

_____

_____

_____

_____

_____

_____

_____

_____

_____

Date:_____ Time:_____

Location: _____

_____

_____

_____

_____

_____

_____

_____

_____

_____

_____

_____

_____

_____

_____

_____

_____

Date:_____ Time:_____

Location: _____

_____

_____

_____

_____

_____

_____

_____

_____

_____

_____

_____

_____

_____

_____

_____

_____

All the peace, wisdom, and joy in the universe are already within us; we don't have to gain, develop, or attain them... We don't need to imagine trees, flowers, deer, birds, and sky; we merely need to open our eyes and realize what is already here, and who we really are.

Date:_____ Time:_____   *Unknown*

Location: _____

_____

_____

_____

_____

_____

_____

_____

_____

_____

_____

_____

_____

_____

_____

When we feel love and kindness toward others, it not only makes others feel loved and cared for, but it helps us also to develop inner happiness and peace.
His Holiness the Dalai Lama

Date:_____ Time:_____

Location: _____

_____

_____

_____

_____

_____

_____

_____

_____

_____

_____

_____

_____

_____

_____

Date:_____ Time:_____

Location: _____

_____

_____

_____

_____

_____

_____

_____

_____

_____

_____

_____

_____

_____

_____

_____

_____

Date:_____ Time:_____

Location: _____
_____
_____
_____
_____
_____
_____
_____
_____
_____
_____
_____
_____
_____
_____
_____
_____
_____

Date:_____ Time:_____

Location: _____

Date:_____ Time:_____

Location: _____

_____

_____

_____

_____

_____

_____

_____

_____

_____

_____

_____

_____

_____

_____

_____

Date:_____ Time:_____

Location: _____

For it isn't enough to talk about peace. One must believe it.
And it isn't enough to believe in it.
One must work at it. —
Eleanor Roosevelt

Date:_____ Time:_____

Location: _____

_____

_____

_____

_____

_____

_____

_____

_____

_____

_____

_____

_____

_____

_____

Responsibility does not only lie with the leaders of our countries . . . It lies with each of us individually. Peace, starts within each one of us. When we have inner peace, we can be at peace with those around us.
His Holiness the Dalai Lama

Date:_____ Time:_____

Location: _____

_____

_____

_____

_____

_____

_____

_____

_____

_____

_____

_____

_____

_____

_____

Date:_____ Time:_____

Location: _____

_____

_____

_____

_____

_____

_____

_____

_____

_____

_____

_____

_____

_____

_____

Date:_____ Time:_____

Location: _____

_____

_____

_____

_____

_____

_____

_____

_____

_____

_____

_____

_____

_____

_____

_____

_____

Date:_____ Time:_____

Location: _____

_____

_____

_____

_____

_____

_____

_____

_____

_____

_____

_____

_____

_____

_____

_____

_____

Date:_____ Time:_____

Location: _____

_____

_____

_____

_____

_____

_____

_____

_____

_____

_____

_____

_____

_____

_____

_____

Date:_____ Time:_____

Location: _____

_____

_____

_____

_____

_____

_____

_____

_____

_____

_____

_____

_____

_____

_____

_____

I keep the telephone of my mind open to peace, harmony, health, love and abundance.
Then whenever doubt, anxiety, or fear try to call me, they keep getting a busy signal
and soon they'll forget my number.
Edith Armstrong

Date:_____ Time:_____

Location: _____

I am the dust in the sunlight, I am the ball of the sun . . .
I am the mist of morning, the breath of evening . . . .
I am the spark in the stone, the gleam of gold in the metal . . . .
The rose and the nightingale drunk with its fragrance.

I am the chain of being, the circle of the spheres,
The scale of creation, the rise and the fall.
I am what is and is not . . .
I am the soul in all.

~ Rumi

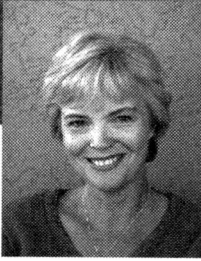

Be Peace Now Audio

with Laurelle Shanti Gaia

Be Peace Now Audio Program
instructions, mantras and chants

We offer audio support for the contents of this manual. The audio program is a guide to help Be Peace Now practitioners develop a deeper understanding of the course.

The program includes a talk on the concepts of the self study course, the symbols, sacred intention, creating sacred space, using affirmations and mantras, and journalling.

Also included are live peace sessions guided by Laurelle, which include the affirmations and chants for;

◆ Establishing the Altea Space

◆ Anchoring the Infinite Light

◆ Divine Alignment

◆ Energizing the Peace Stream

Also included is a nine minute Om Shanti Gaia chanting session, which can be used to support your meditations, or to help energize your home, or work space, while providing energetic support for all peace weavers. A nine minute crystal bowl sound session is included, as well as a drumming session for grounding and anchoring the energy.

To order visit www.BePeaceNow.com or call 800-359-3424 or 928-204-1216
The price of the Be Peace Now Audio Program is $44

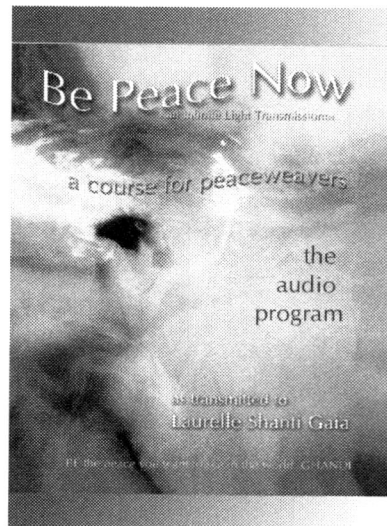

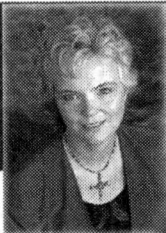

CD Journeys with Laurelle Shanti Gaia

Infinite Spectrum 8 Chakra Journey

Journey into the healing power of your soul using color, light and sound. Laurelle Gaia gently guides this healing journey on CD, that contains a 45 minute color energy session which can be used for relaxation, self empowerment and also used with clients.

Listen to this beautiful healing experience time and time again, and it can help you in new ways everytime you participate in it.

Includes CD, booklet and affirmation cards.
ISBN 0-9678721-1-1 $29.55

Sacred Circles... Journey into the angelic realms and inner planes

Recorded LIVE at the Annual International Reiki Retreat.

Introducing The Sacred Circle and the Ascension Ring. Manifestation tools for aligning with the Divine and awakenting to peace.

Learn to soul link with other lightworkers, Reiki guides and angels. Includes CD, booklet and affirmation cards. UPC 634479260421 $29.95

We are currently developing Reiki Review CDs, Reiki meditations and many more self development programs. Watch our online store for new releases www.ReikiClasses.com
To order call us toll free 1-800-359-3424 or send an email to IamInfiniteLight@aol.com or visit www.InfiniteLight.com

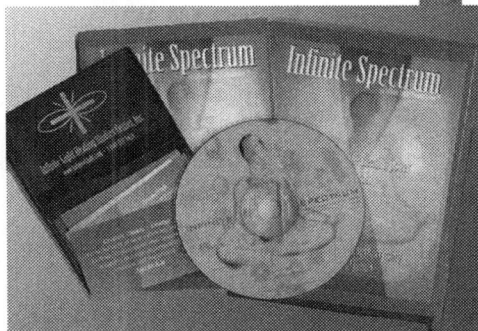

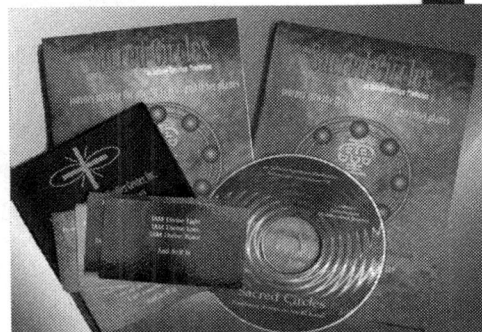

Seminars & Sessions in Sacred & Magical Sedona, Arizona

with Laurelle Shanti Gaia & Michael Arthur Baird

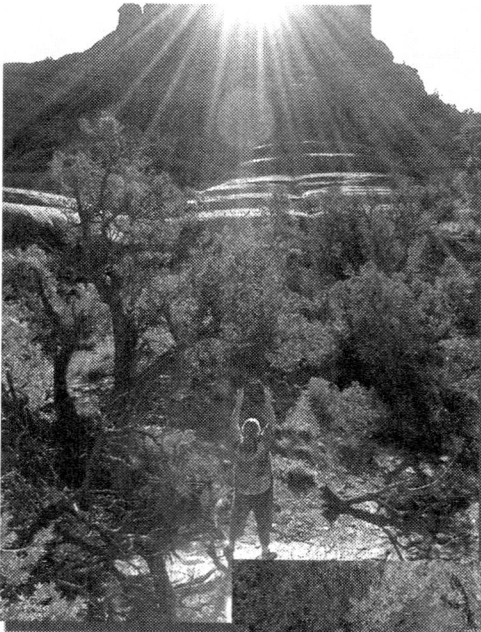

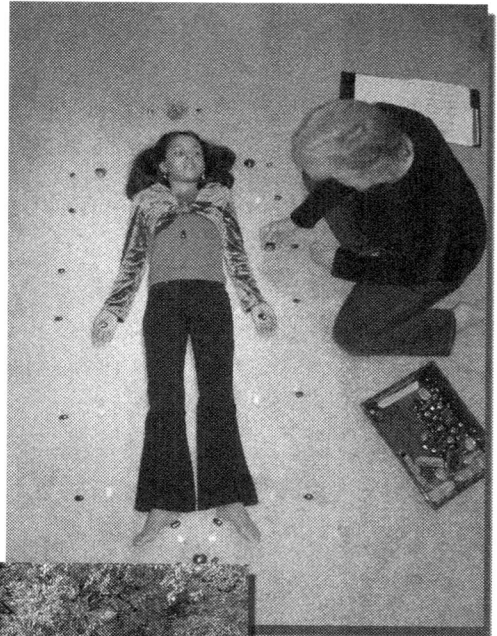

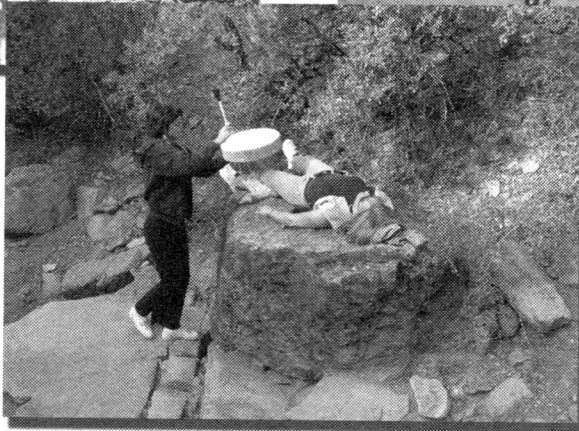

Infinite Light, Peaceweaving, Sound Healing,
Reiki Crystal Healing, Color Healing,
Reiki Drumming, Usui Reiki, Usui Tibetan Reiki,
Karuna Reiki®

Imagine there's no heaven, It's easy if you try,
No hell below us, Above us only sky,
Imagine all the people living for today...

Imagine there's no countries, It isnt hard to do,
Nothing to kill or die for, No religion too,
Imagine all the people living life in peace...

Imagine no possesions, I wonder if you can,
No need for greed or hunger, A brotherhood of man,
Imagine all the peopleSharing all the world...

You may say Im a dreamer, but Im not the only one,
I hope some day you'll join us,
And the world will live as one.

John Lennon

www.ingramcontent.com/pod-product-compliance
Lightning Source LLC
Chambersburg PA
CBHW080334270326
41927CB00014B/3212